FITNESS BOOST FOR SENIORS:

HOLISTIC WORKOUTS FOR SENIORS FOR WEIGHT LOSS, STRENGTH, AND ENHANCED FLEXIBILITY

BAILEY BLAKE

CONTENTS

INTRODUCTION

Understanding The Importance Of Senior Fitness

In the tapestry of life, where every thread weaves the tale of our journey, the relevance of senior fitness appears as a brilliant and transformational hue. As we gracefully embrace the golden chapters of our lives, the resonance of a well-crafted fitness routine reverberates across the physical, mental, and emotional components of our well-being.

A Symphony of Physical Health: Picture the heart as the conductor directing the beat of life. Through the artistry of regular exercise, we strengthen our hearts, producing cardiovascular health that transcends the ticking of time. Aerobic exercises, like a musical crescendo, boost blood circulation, dance with the rhythms of longevity, and create a harmonic symphony of well-being.

In the dance of bones and joints, we reveal the subtle choreography of preserving strength and flexibility. Weight-bearing exercises and the beautiful dance of resistance training build a masterpiece that fortifies bones, leaving an unmistakable imprint on the canvas of joint health, avoiding the shadows of osteoporosis and maintaining the fluidity of movement.

The Art of Balance: Weight regulation, a delicate brushstroke in the image of senior fitness, enables us to explore the canvas of our bodies. A well-constructed fitness regimen becomes the paintbrush, helping us to draw the outlines of a healthy weight, sheltering us from the storm of obesity-related diseases. It is a canvas where strokes of purpose generate a masterpiece of well-managed vibrancy.

Cognitive Flourish: The cognitive theater of our thoughts unfurls as we explore into the cognitive advantages conferred by a physically active lifestyle. The scene is prepared for a mental show, where exercise becomes the protagonist, increasing brain health, promoting memory retention, and minimizing the shadows of cognitive decline. Each session is a standing ovation for a mind that refuses to submit to the passage of time.

Emotional Resonance: The emotional landscape emerges as we explore the vast garden of senior fitness. Stress, that discordant note in life's symphony, finds resolution in the peaceful tones of regular exercise. The mood, enhanced by the endorphins, those celestial notes of joy, ascends, contrasting the shadows of despair with a song of well-being.

Social Connection: In the complex tapestry of emotional well-being, the social thread weaves its complicated pattern. Senior fitness isn't only a solo endeavor but a community celebration. Group activities, workshops, and community participation construct a sonnet of social connection, easing the loneliness that may throw shadows on our emotional landscape.

The Tapestry of Independence: Enhanced everyday functionality becomes the brushstroke that paints the hues of independence. Strength, balance, and flexibility, the hues on the palette, unite to produce a masterpiece that allows us to relish in the autonomy of our daily lives, each stroke contributing to the rich tapestry of our life.

A Symphony for a Longer Overture: Finally, we investigate the notion of active aging, where exercise becomes the screenplay for a longer and more vibrant existence. The trip is not only about counting the years but about ensuring that each year is a celebration, a monument to the enduring spirit that refuses to be restricted by age.

Overview of the Holistic Approach

In the broad fabric of life, the golden years call us to take a comprehensive approach to health. "Fitness Boost for Seniors: Holistic Workouts for seniors for Weight Loss, Strength, and Enhanced Flexibility" is not only a guide; it's an invitation to go on a transforming adventure. This chapter emerges like a compass, directing seniors toward a holistic fitness paradigm that supports the body, mind, and spirit.

The Essence of Holistic Fitness:

At its foundation, holistic fitness transcends the usual constraints of workout regimes. It is a strategy that respects the complicated interplay of physical, mental, and emotional well-being. In our research, we shall expose the multiple layers of this holistic approach, discovering how each component adds to a symphony of health that echoes through every fiber of our life.

Physical Vitality:

Our journey begins with the physical vitality that is the cornerstone of comprehensive wellness. Rather of considering exercise as a mundane necessity, we embrace it as a celebration of movement. Holistic exercises for seniors aren't about rigorous routines; they're a choreography of thoughtful movements, meant to boost cardiovascular health, develop joint flexibility, and sculpt lean muscle.

In the search of weight loss, we unlock the secrets of a balanced diet, perceiving nutrition not as a limiting idea but as a partner in our path toward vitality. The chapter unveils the art of mindful eating, providing light on the tremendous influence of nutrition on our energy levels, metabolism, and general well-being.

Mental Fortitude:

The second phase of our comprehensive inquiry dives into the domain of mental fortitude. We realize that the mind is not a separate entity but an intrinsic aspect of our entire being. Cognitive function becomes our canvas, and exercise the brush that paints strokes of clarity and insight.

Stress, the hidden opponent of mental well-being, is handled not just as a symptom but as a chance for resilience. The holistic approach argues for stress management approaches interwoven throughout our workout routines, promoting mental resilience via activities such as mindfulness and meditation.

Emotional Resilience:

Emotional well-being unfurls like a garden inside the holistic environment. Here, we study the emotional resonance of fitness, where exercise becomes a therapeutic method. We acknowledge the influence of endorphins, those delightful molecules of joy, on our emotional state. By embracing group activities and community participation, we cultivate the seeds of social connection, creating emotional resilience in the rich soil of shared experiences.

Integration of Holistic Workouts:

The chapter then easily moves into the practical incorporation of holistic training. Rather of giving a fixed framework, we give a palette of possibilities customized to individual interests and skills. From energizing yoga sessions that mix physical activity with mental peace to dynamic strength training routines that shape and strengthen, the holistic approach suits varied tastes.

Mind-Body Synchrony:

Holistic fitness is not a disconnected collection of activities but a symphony of mind and body synchronicity. We explore the notion of mindful movement, where each activity is a chance to connect with our body. Through guided breathing and conscious mindfulness, we establish a stronger link between our physical acts and mental state, boosting the total impact of our exercises.

Celebrating Progress:

Within the holistic approach, progress is not judged merely by bodily modifications but by the milestones attained in mental clarity, emotional resilience, and the joy obtained from the trip. The chapter gives an invitation to enjoy each step forward, understanding that holistic health is a lifetime trip with no fixed goal.

A Lifestyle, Not a Task:

Crucially, holistic fitness is not an isolated chore but a lifestyle embraced with joy. It infiltrates every element of our daily routine, from the meals we pick to the beliefs we create. The chapter urges seniors to consider exercise not as a stressful responsibility but as a dynamic, rewarding lifestyle that promotes lifespan, quality of life, and the simple joy of living.

CHAPTER 1

GETTING STATRTED

Assessing Fitness Levels

In the road toward holistic wellness, recognizing where we stand becomes the compass directing our route. "Fitness Boost for Seniors: Holistic Workouts for Seniors for Weight Loss, Strength, and Enhanced Flexibility" recognizes that each senior embarks on a unique path, and assessing fitness levels is the cornerstone of tailoring a wellness journey that suits individual capabilities, aspirations, and health considerations.

The Holistic Perspective:

Before diving into the mechanics of fitness testing, it's necessary to build a comprehensive picture. Fitness isn't a one-dimensional characteristic defined just by physical skills; it's a tapestry woven with strands of physical vitality, mental sharpness, and emotional fortitude. Therefore, our evaluation paradigm stretches beyond typical fitness indicators, incorporating a holistic grasp of the individual's well-being.

Physical Fitness Assessment:

Cardiovascular Endurance:

We began our fitness examination with cardiovascular endurance, often called the pulse of holistic wellbeing. Simple examinations like quick walking or stepping exercises determine how well the heart and lungs interact, offering insights into the body's ability to maintain aerobic activity.

Muscular Strength and Endurance:

The examination then switches to the world of musculoskeletal strength and endurance. We participate in resistance exercises suited to individual capacities, testing the capacity to apply force and tolerate sustained muscular activation. This component is crucial, especially in developing routines that improve strength while limiting weariness or injury.

Flexibility and Joint Mobility:

The fluidity of movement is studied through examinations of

flexibility and joint mobility. Yoga-inspired stretches and joint exercises unravel the body's range of motion, delivering useful insights into regions that may require concentrated attention. Flexibility tests also aid to the avoidance of accidents and the promotion of general mobility.

Mental and Cognitive Fitness Assessment:

Cognitive Function:

Our complete examination extends to the cognitive sphere. Engaging in mental tasks that test memory, attention, and problem-solving abilities gives a window into cognitive function. This dimension highlights the interdependence of physical and mental well-being, emphasizing that a keen mind is as vital as a healthy body.

Stress Resilience and Emotional Well-being:

Emotional resilience and stress management are measured through guided mindfulness activities. Seniors are encouraged to reflect on their stress coping techniques, building a knowledge of emotional well-being. This evaluation emphasizes the substantial effect of emotional health on overall fitness and lays the scene for individualized stress-relief measures within holistic exercises.

Lifestyle and Well-being Assessment:

Nutritional Analysis:

Nutrition, a vital part of holistic wellbeing, is evaluated through a nutritional analysis. Seniors are urged to reflect on eating habits, finding areas of improvement and fostering an understanding of the symbiotic link between nutrition and exercise. This evaluation creates the framework for tailored nutritional recommendations that complement comprehensive exercises.

Sleep Patterns:

An often-overlooked component of well-being, sleep habits, is brought into light. Seniors analyze the quality and length of their sleep, acknowledging the function of rest in the healing and rejuvenation process. This feature adds to the construction of holistic workouts that correspond with circadian cycles, enhancing the effects of both exercise and sleep.

Social Engagement and Support:

Social connections, vital for emotional well-being, are examined through an examination of social engagement and support networks. Seniors reflect on their social connections, discovering chances for community participation within their fitness journey. This examination encourages the awareness that holistic fitness extends beyond individual efforts, thriving within the embrace of a supportive community.

Interpreting Fitness Assessment Results:

The assessment step culminates with a nuanced interpretation of outcomes. Rather of presenting outcomes as fixed judgments, we regard them as dynamic beginning places, moving seniors toward areas that demand attention and celebration. The holistic approach allows seniors to celebrate development not only in physical achievements but also in cognitive sharpness, emotional resilience, and the subtle adjustments inside their lifestyle.

Crafting a Personalized Fitness Journey:

Armed with a comprehensive grasp of their fitness environment, seniors are now set to embark on a tailored fitness journey. The comprehensive exercises given in later chapters become personalized creations, adjusted to correspond with individual objectives, tastes, and health considerations.

Setting Realistic Goals

In the kaleidoscope of senior wellness, setting realistic objectives emerges as the compass leading the transforming path covered in "Fitness Boost for Seniors: Holistic Workouts for Seniors for Weight Loss, Strength, and Enhanced Flexibility." This chapter emerges as a guide, directing seniors through the difficult landscape of goal-setting, assuring that each step is not merely doable but profoundly satisfying.

The Essence of Realistic Goals:

At the center of our investigation lies a fundamental truth: sustained growth is created from realistic goals. In a world that typically extols fast transitions, we redefine success within the framework of senior fitness. Realism becomes the cornerstone, allowing seniors to create milestones that reflect individual capabilities, reward growth, and encourage a sense of achievement at every level.

Understanding Individual Baselines:

The trip begins with a thorough dive into individual baselines. Before going on the path of goal-setting, seniors engage in a careful contemplation on their existing fitness levels. We acknowledge that each senior is a unique canvas, painted with particular experiences, health issues, and goals. The chapter calls for a comprehensive examination that incorporates physical, mental, and emotional components, creating a framework for objectives that fit with individual beginning points.

Physical Realism:

Cardiovascular Endurance:

For individuals wanting to better cardiovascular health, realism emerges in modest increases. Seniors create objectives based on attainable periods of brisk walking or low-impact aerobics, acknowledging the body's response to increasing exercise. The emphasis is not on the distance traveled but on the constancy of effort, developing a sustainable rhythm.

Muscular Strength and Endurance:

Realistic strength objectives reflect the individuality of each senior's muscular potential. Rather of fixating on lifting large weights, the focus changes to resistance training that progressively pushes muscles while minimizing strain. Seniors appreciate tiny increases in repetitions, providing a sense of empowerment anchored on attainable success.

Flexibility and Joint Mobility:

Flexibility objectives resonate with the body's natural range of motion. Seniors establish reasonable aims in stretching programs, understanding that flexibility increases gradually. The chapter promotes a conscious exploration of yoga-inspired motions, appreciating the delight of greater mobility rather than fixating on severe contortions.

Mental and Cognitive Realism:

Cognitive Function:

Realistic objectives in cognitive fitness respect the mind's existing condition. Seniors engage in mental activities that challenge memory and problem-solving abilities at a speed that fosters achievement. The chapter underlines the significance of consistency, viewing cognitive training as a marathon rather than a sprint.

Stress Resilience and Emotional Well-being:

Emotional health goals are founded on stress management practices that match with individual preferences. Seniors pursue practical stress-relief strategies such as mindfulness, realizing that emotional resilience is created via moderate, regular efforts. The focus is on establishing a toolset of coping techniques rather than expecting instantaneous transformation.

Lifestyle and Well-being Realism:

Nutritional Adjustments:

Nutrition objectives incorporate a practical approach to dietary modifications. Seniors establish attainable targets, whether it's integrating more fruits and vegetables or maintaining water levels. Realism becomes the base, knowing that sustained nutritional adjustments are gradual, allowing for an easier incorporation into daily life.

Sleep Patterns:

Realistic sleep objectives focus the quality of slumber above immediate adjustments. Seniors adopt practices that encourage greater sleep hygiene, knowing that gains may emerge incrementally. The chapter highlights that sleep is not a goal but a continuous part of overall well-being.

Social Engagement and Support:

Social connection aims honor individual comfort levels. Seniors establish reasonable aims for community involvement, realizing that the route toward social engagement is a personal experience. The focus is on generating possibilities for interaction rather than complying to external expectations.

The Nuances of Progress:

Realistic objectives accept the intricacies of growth. Seniors are taught to evaluate success not just via measurable measurements but as a tapestry woven with various achievements. The chapter redefines success within the framework of holistic well-being, highlighting the delight obtained from constant effort and the celebration of milestones that may not be evident on typical fitness monitors.

Goal Adjustments and Adaptability:

The chapter instills an attitude of adaptation. Seniors learn that goal-setting is not a strict contract but a dynamic dialogue with their changing selves. The wisdom is in the flexibility to change goals based on changing circumstances, health considerations, and personal preferences. Adaptability becomes a tribute to resilience and self-awareness.

Fostering a Sense of Accomplishment:

In our investigation of realistic goal-setting, a vital theme emerges – the creation of a strong sense of accomplishment. Seniors are not only participants in a workout regimen; they are architects of their overall well-being. Each realistic objective becomes a stepping stone, not simply toward physical milestones but, more crucially, toward a persistent sensation of empowerment and energy.

Creating a Personalized Workout Plan

In the dynamic landscape of senior fitness, the chapter on designing a personalized workout plan emerges like a compass, directing each individual toward a bespoke journey of holistic wellbeing. *"Fitness Boost for Seniors: Holistic Workouts for Seniors for Weight Loss, Strength, and Enhanced Flexibility"* embraces the individuality of every senior, realizing that a one-size-fits-all strategy is not only unrealistic but counterproductive. This part of chapter 1 is an invitation to develop a fitness story that connects with personal objectives, interests, and the intricate fabric of individual well-being.

Understanding Your Body:

Before digging into the complexities of a tailored training regimen, we go on a voyage of self-discovery. Understanding one's body becomes the core pillar of holistic fitness. Seniors engage in gentle self-assessments, examining how their body responds to various motions, finding areas of strength, and highlighting zones that may require concentrated attention. This introspective phase creates the framework for a fitness routine that corresponds flawlessly with individual capabilities.

Tailoring Cardiovascular Exercises:

Brisk Walking and Low-Impact Aerobics:

For seniors adopting the road of cardiovascular health, the individualized strategy begins with the moderate tempo of brisk walking. The charm resides in its simplicity; it is a kind of exercise that suits varied fitness levels. Seniors establish reasonable objectives for daily steps, gradually increasing the time and intensity of walks. Low-impact aerobics, embellished with pleasant motions, offer an option that keeps the heart engaged without exerting undue stress on joints.

Cycling and Swimming:

The individualized plan grows to incorporate alternatives such as cycling and swimming. These low-impact workouts harness the therapeutic potential of buoyancy, supporting cardiovascular health while enjoying the fluidity of motion. Seniors pick activities that resonate with their interests, injecting joy into the road toward greater heart health.

Building Muscular Strength and Endurance:

Resistance Training using Light Weights:

The road toward physical strength and endurance unfolds with resistance training utilizing small weights. The tailored plan provides a series of workouts targeting main muscle groups. Seniors engage in bicep curls, leg lifts, and sitting rows, nurturing strength without the strain. The emphasis is on controlled motions that empower rather than exhaust.

Bodyweight Exercises:

Bodyweight exercises become a vital element of the individualized regimen, knowing that the body itself is a potent instrument for gaining strength. Seniors experience squats, lunges, and modified push-ups, progressively developing based on individual comfort levels. The beauty of bodyweight workouts resides in their flexibility to various fitness stages.

Enhancing Flexibility with Mindful Movements:

Yoga-Inspired Stretches:

Flexibility takes center stage with yoga-inspired stretches. Seniors engage in a series of mild positions that increase flexibility and joint mobility. The individualized plan emphasizes attentive movements, stressing the relationship between breath and stretch. Each stance becomes a celebration of mobility, encouraging a sense of fluidity in daily activities.

Tai Chi with Qi Gong:

The comprehensive approach extends to incorporate the graceful arts of Tai Chi and Qi Gong. These practices mix movement, breath, and meditation, developing flexibility while cultivating a sense of balance and peace. Seniors blend these ancient disciplines into their individual strategy, embracing the harmonious flow of energy throughout their bodies.

Mindful Cognitive Exercises:

Brain-Boosting Games and Puzzles:

Cognitive fitness plays a key part in the individualized strategy. Seniors participate in brain-boosting games and puzzles that challenge memory, concentration, and problem-solving abilities. The strategy converts cognitive workouts into delightful pastimes, realizing that mental exercises are as crucial to well-being as physical ones.

Mindfulness Meditation:

The individualized strategy integrates mindfulness meditation as a technique for stress reduction and cognitive clarity. Seniors engage on a voyage of self-awareness, discovering guided meditation methods that create a calm and focused mind. Mindfulness becomes not only an exercise but a period of contemplation and renewal.

Nutrition and Hydration Integration:

Balanced Nutrition:

Holistic fitness extends beyond exercise to incorporate nutrition. The individualized plan includes instructions for appropriate eating, knowing that fuelling the body is as crucial as the activities themselves. Seniors explore the vibrant spectrum of fruits, vegetables, lean meats, and healthy grains, establishing a synergy between sustenance and activity.

Hydration Practices:

Hydration becomes a cornerstone of the tailored strategy. Seniors are urged to adopt hydration programs that match their training schedules. The chapter underlines the symbiotic link between appropriate water intake and the body's capacity to perform adequately during activities.

Social Connection and Support:

Group Classes and Community participation: Recognizing the relevance of social connection, the individualized approach integrates group classes and community participation. Seniors pursue local exercise programs or virtual groups that accord with their interests. Whether it's a dancing class, a walking club, or an online fitness network, the plan celebrates the companionship that generates motivation and support.

Celebrating Progress and Adaptability:

The chapter highlights the necessity of recognizing progress within the individualized plan. Seniors are taught to regard each milestone, whether great or small, as a win. Progress becomes a dynamic interaction with one's changing self, and flexibility becomes a fundamental characteristic. The plan understands that adaptations may be necessary based on health considerations, and it gives advise on adapting workouts to match with changing conditions.

CHAPTER 2

WEIGHT LOSS
STRATEGIES

Nutrition Tips for Seniors

Healthy and lean living in retirement requires a detailed dietary plan customized to seniors' requirements. Beyond counting calories, this weight reduction path transforms into a purposeful acceptance of nutritional meals that boost energy, strength, and well-being.

The enlightening "Fitness Boost for Seniors: Holistic Workouts for Seniors for Weight Loss, Strength, and Enhanced Flexibility," provides a persuasive guidance. Not merely a guidebook, this guide is a roadmap for seniors, providing a comprehensive plan to manage weight through strategic and pleasant diet.

Knowing Nutrient-Dense Options:

Exploring nutritional density starts the adventure. Seniors should focus on vitamin-, mineral-, and nutrient-rich meals to maximize every bite. This is a purposeful effort to make every calorie count and support the body's processes while enjoying a variety of healthy foods.

Macronutrient Balance:

Protein, carbohydrate, and fat balance is key. Seniors dive into the relevance of combining lean proteins for muscle maintenance, complex carbs for sustained energy, and healthy fats for satiety. The objective extends beyond nutritional balance; it's about producing meals that are not simply healthful but also pleasing to the senses.

Portion Control and Mindful Eating:

Portion control becomes a vital factor as seniors master the ability of listening to their body and practicing mindful eating. The book recommends enjoying each mouthful, acknowledging the subtle indications of hunger and fullness. Through adopting a mindful attitude to eating, weight management changes into a conscious and joyful experience rather than a rigid schedule.

Hydration for Weight Loss Support:

Hydration appears as a sturdy ally in the weight reduction path. Seniors reveal the significance of water in increasing satiety and maintaining metabolic functioning. Practical ideas are presented to promote regular hydration, making water into a delightful and crucial component of their weight reduction approach.

Embracing Fiber-Rich Foods:

The guide enthusiastically advocates for the inclusion of fiber-rich foods as steadfast champions in the struggle for weight loss. Seniors embark on a voyage through fruits, vegetables, whole grains, and legumes, knowing how fiber creates a sensation of fullness and supports in digestive health. This is not simply a weight reduction trip; it's a route towards sustainable and nutritious weight control.

Lean Proteins for Muscle Preservation:

The tale unveils the crucial significance of lean proteins in the weight reduction journey—not simply for losing pounds but for sustaining essential muscle mass. Seniors explore a varied variety of protein sources, from poultry and fish to plant-based alternatives, constructing meals that assist weight loss without compromising strength.

Smart Snacking Strategies:

Snacking receives a redefinition, evolving into a purposeful and pleasurable component of the weight loss plan. Seniors find clever snacking alternatives that offer energy between meals without derailing progress. The book enables the investigation of healthful snacks harmonizing with individual preferences and dietary needs.

Meal Planning for Success:

Seniors are equipped with meal planning methods supporting success on the weight loss path. The guide unveils the art of preparing balanced meals in advance, so each day is full with nutritional choices. This practical strategy converts weight control from a daunting undertaking into a smooth and doable lifestyle.

The Role of Physical Activity in Weight Loss:

Physical exercise plays a crucial function as a supplementary factor in weight loss. Seniors obtain insights on how a well-rounded physical regimen increases the efficiency of their eating plan. The guide gives practical information on pre- and post-workout nutrition, highlighting the symbiotic link between exercise and nutritional choices.

Celebrating Progress and Enjoying the Journey:

The weight reduction journey transcends the goal; it's a celebration of progress and a commitment to sustained lifestyle improvements. Seniors are not merely encouraged but exhorted to celebrate milestones, realizing that each step toward their weight loss objectives is an accomplishment. The guide develops a positive mentality, ensuring the journey is not just productive but pleasant and powerful. This isn't only a guide—it's an invitation for seniors to begin on a transforming path towards a healthier, leaner, and more vibrant self.

The enlightening "Fitness Boost for Seniors: Holistic Workouts for Seniors for Weight Loss, Strength, and Enhanced Flexibility," provides a persuasive guidance. Not merely a guidebook, this guide is a roadmap for seniors, providing a comprehensive plan to manage weight through strategic and pleasant diet.

Knowing Nutrient-Dense Options:

Exploring nutritional density starts the adventure. Seniors should focus on vitamin-, mineral-, and nutrient-rich meals to maximize every bite. This is a purposeful effort to make every calorie count and support the body's processes while enjoying a variety of healthy foods.

Macronutrient Balance:

Protein, carbohydrate, and fat balance is key. Seniors dive into the relevance of combining lean proteins for muscle maintenance, complex carbs for sustained energy, and healthy fats for satiety. The objective extends beyond nutritional balance; it's about producing meals that are not simply healthful but also pleasing to the senses.

Portion Control and Mindful Eating:

Portion control becomes a vital factor as seniors master the ability of listening to their body and practicing mindful eating. The book recommends enjoying each mouthful, acknowledging the subtle indications of hunger and fullness. Through adopting a mindful attitude to eating, weight management changes into a conscious and joyful experience rather than a rigid schedule.

Hydration for Weight Loss Support:

Hydration appears as a sturdy ally in the weight reduction path. Seniors reveal the significance of water in increasing satiety and maintaining metabolic functioning. Practical ideas are presented to promote regular hydration, making water into a delightful and crucial component of their weight reduction approach.

Embracing Fiber-Rich Foods:

The guide enthusiastically advocates for the inclusion of fiber-rich foods as steadfast champions in the struggle for weight loss. Seniors embark on a voyage through fruits, vegetables, whole grains, and legumes, knowing how fiber creates a sensation of fullness and supports in digestive health. This is not simply a weight reduction trip; it's a route towards sustainable and nutritious weight control.

Lean Proteins for Muscle Preservation:

The tale unveils the crucial significance of lean proteins in the weight reduction journey—not simply for losing pounds but for sustaining essential muscle mass. Seniors explore a varied variety of protein sources, from poultry and fish to plant-based alternatives, constructing meals that assist weight loss without compromising strength.

Smart Snacking Strategies:

Snacking receives a redefinition, evolving into a purposeful and pleasurable component of the weight loss plan. Seniors find clever snacking alternatives that offer energy between meals without derailing progress. The book enables the investigation of healthful snacks harmonizing with individual preferences and dietary needs.

Meal Planning for Success:

Seniors are equipped with meal planning methods supporting success on the weight loss path. The guide unveils the art of preparing balanced meals in advance, so each day is full with nutritional choices. This practical strategy converts weight control from a daunting undertaking into a smooth and doable lifestyle.

The Role of Physical Activity in Weight Loss:

Physical exercise plays a crucial function as a supplementary factor in weight loss. Seniors obtain insights on how a well-rounded physical regimen increases the efficiency of their eating plan. The guide gives practical information on pre- and post-workout nutrition, highlighting the symbiotic link between exercise and nutritional choices.

Celebrating Progress and Enjoying the Journey:

The weight reduction journey transcends the goal; it's a celebration of progress and a commitment to sustained lifestyle improvements. Seniors are not merely encouraged but exhorted to celebrate milestones, realizing that each step toward their weight loss objectives is an accomplishment. The guide develops a positive mentality, ensuring the journey is not just productive but pleasant and powerful. This isn't only a guide—it's an invitation for seniors to begin on a transforming path towards a healthier, leaner, and more vibrant self.

Effective Cardio Workouts For Weight Management

As seniors embark on their fitness journey, incorporating effective cardio workouts becomes paramount for weight management. These exercises not only promote cardiovascular health but also aid in burning calories, contributing to weight loss and overall well-being. Below are some tailored cardio workouts for seniors, along with recommended sets and repetitions.

Walking or Brisk Walking:

Sets: 3-4 sets

Repetitions: 15-30 minutes per set

Gentle yet effective, walking is an ideal low-impact cardio exercise for seniors. Begin with a moderate pace and gradually increase intensity. Aim for 3-4 sets, with each set lasting 15-30 minutes, depending on individual fitness levels.

Cycling:

Sets: 3 sets

Repetitions: 10-20 minutes per set

Cycling, whether on a stationary bike or outdoors, offers a joint-friendly cardio option. Seniors can start with 3 sets, cycling at a comfortable pace for 10-20 minutes per set. Adjust resistance based on fitness levels.

Swimming or Water Aerobics:

Sets: 2-3 sets

Repetitions: 20-30 minutes per set

Water-based exercises are gentle on joints. Engage in swimming or water aerobics for 2-3 sets, with each set lasting 20-30 minutes. The resistance of water enhances the workout's effectiveness.

Dancing:

Sets: 2-3 sets

Repetitions: 15-30 minutes per set

Dancing is a fun way to stay active. Opt for dance styles that suit individual preferences. Aim for 2-3 dance sessions, with each session lasting 15-30 minutes. It's an enjoyable way to boost heart rate and burn calories.

Elliptical Training:

Sets: 3 sets

Repetitions: 10-15 minutes per set

The elliptical machine provides a low-impact, full-body workout. Seniors can start with 3 sets, each lasting 10-15 minutes. Adjust resistance and incline as needed for an effective workout.

Seated Exercises:

Sets: 2-3 sets

Repetitions: 15-20 minutes per set

Seated exercises are ideal for those with limited mobility. Engage in seated leg lifts, arm circles, or seated marching. Aim for 2-3 sets, with each set lasting 15-20 minutes.

Stationary Marching:

Sets: 3-4 sets

Repetitions: 15-20 minutes per set Stationary marching is a convenient option. Lift the knees while standing in place. Aim for 3-4 sets, with each set lasting 15-20 minutes. It's an effective way to elevate the heart rate.Stationary marching is a convenient option. Lift the knees while standing in place. Aim for 3-4 sets, with each set lasting 15-20 minutes. It's an effective way to elevate the heart rate.

Chair Exercises:

Sets: 2-3 sets

Repetitions: 15-20 minutes per set

Chair workouts are adaptable and can be adapted to individual needs. Seated marches, seated leg lifts, or seated toe taps can be included. Aim for 2-3 sets, with each set lasting 15-20 minutes. These exercises are mild on the joints and appropriate for persons with restricted mobility.

Tai Chi:

Sets: Continuous flow

Repetitions: 20-30 minutes

Tai Chi blends soft, flowing motions with deep breathing, developing balance, flexibility, and relaxation. Seniors can engage in continuous Tai Chi sessions, aiming for 20-30 minutes. It increases cardiovascular health while focusing on mindfulness.

Stair Climbing:

Sets: 3 sets

Repetitions: 5-10 minutes per set

Climbing stairs is an efficient strategy to boost the heart rate. For elders, this can be done on a staircase at home or on a stair-climbing machine. Start with 3 sets, ascending for 5-10 minutes per set. It's a practical and accessible cardio program.

Resistance Band Aerobics:

Sets: 2-3 sets

Repetitions: 15-20 minutes per set

Incorporating resistance bands adds a strength element to cardio. Seniors can practice activities like seated rowing or standing side steps with resistance bands. Aim for 2-3 sets, with each session lasting 15-20 minutes, focusing on controlled movements.

Rowing Machine:

Sets: 3 sets

Repetitions: 10-15 minutes per set

Rowing gives a full-body workout without putting excessive strain on joints. Utilize a rowing machine for 3 sets, rowing for 10-15 minutes every set. It promotes cardiovascular fitness while activating main muscle groups.

Mini Trampoline (Rebounding):

Sets: 2-3 sets

Repetitions: 10-15 minutes per set

Rebounding on a tiny trampoline is a low-impact yet efficient cardio exercise. Seniors can bounce gently for 2-3 sets, with each set lasting 10-15 minutes. It enhances balance, coordination, and cardiovascular health.

Pilates: Sets: Continuous flow

Repetitions: 20-30 minutes

Pilates focuses on core strength, flexibility, and controlled movements. Seniors can engage in continuous Pilates exercises, aiming for 20-30 minutes. It increases general fitness and may be tailored to various fitness levels.

Elliptical Trainer with Handles:

Sets: 3 sets

Repetitions: 10-15 minutes per set

Using an elliptical machine with handles adds an upper body

workout to the cardio regimen. Seniors can start with 3 sets, exercising for 10-15 minutes per set. It's a low-impact choice that develops cardiovascular endurance.

Gardening Cardio: Sets: Continuous activity

Repetitions: 30-45 minutes

Gardening exercises, such as raking, digging, or vigorous walking while gardening, might help to cardiovascular health. Seniors can engage in continuous gardening for 30-45 minutes, enjoying the outdoors while being active.

Chapter 3

BUILDING STRENGTH RESISTANCE TRAINING FOR SENIORS

Legs (Quadriceps, Hamstrings, Calves):

Exercise: Bodyweight Squats

Description: Stand with feet shoulder-width apart. Lower your body by bending at the knees and hips, as if sitting back into an imaginary chair. Keep your back straight and chest up. Lower until thighs are parallel to the ground, then push through your heels to return to the starting position.

Arms (Biceps, Triceps):

Exercise: Bicep Curls with Light Weights

Description: Hold a light weight in each hand, arms fully stretched at your sides. Slowly lift the weights toward your shoulders, maintaining your elbows tight to your torso. Lower the weights back down with control. This targets the biceps.

Chest (Pectoral Muscles):

Exercise: Wall Push-Ups

Description: Stand facing a wall at arm's length. Place your hands on the wall at shoulder height. Lower your chest towards the wall by bending your elbows, then push back to the starting position. This workout focuses the chest.

Back (Latissimus Dorsi):

Exercise: Seated Rows with Resistance Band Description: Sit on a chair with a resistance band fastened in front. Hold the band with arms extended, palms facing each other. Pull the band towards your chest, pressing your shoulder blades together. Return to the starting position.

Shoulders (Deltoids):

Exercise: Lateral Raises with Light Weights

Description: Hold a light weight in each hand, arms by your sides. Lift the weights out to the sides until they reach shoulder height, then lower them back down with control. This targets the deltoid muscles.

Core (Abdominals, Lower Back):

Exercise: Seated Leg Lifts

Description: Sit on a chair with feet flat on the floor. Lift one leg straight out in front of you, hold for a bit, then lower it back down. Alternate legs. This workout engages the abdominal muscles.

Hips (Glutes):

Exercise: Glute Bridges

Description: Lie on your back with knees bent and feet flat on the floor. Lift your hips towards the ceiling, forming a straight line from shoulders to knees. Squeeze your glutes at the top, then lower back down.

Balance (Legs, Core):

Exercise: One-Leg Stand

Description: Stand near a firm surface for support if needed. Lift one leg off the ground and hold the position for as long as comfortable. Switch to the opposite leg. This exercise promotes balance.

Legs (Quadriceps, Hamstrings, Calves):

Exercise: Standing Calf Raises

Description: Stand with feet hip-width apart. Rise up onto your toes, lifting your heels off the ground. Lower your heels back down to the beginning position. This targets the calf muscles.

Arms (Forearms, Grip Strength):

Exercise: Forearm Squeezes with a Stress Ball Description: Hold a stress ball in one hand and squeeze it strongly, then release. Repeat with the opposite hand. This workout enhances forearm strength and grip.

Chest (Pectoral Muscles): Exercise: Chest Press with Resistance Band

Description: Secure a resistance band to a solid anchor. Hold the band with both hands, arms extended in front. Push the band away from your chest, then return to the beginning position.

Back (Rhomboids): Exercise: Seated Band Pull-Apart

Description: Sit in a chair with a resistance band in front. Hold the band with both hands, arms outstretched. Pull the band apart, pulling your shoulder blades together, then return to the beginning position.

Shoulders (Rotator Cuff): Exercise: Rotator Cuff External Rotation

Description: Hold a small resistance band with one end fixed at waist height. Stand sideways to the band, grasp it with one hand, and rotate your arm outward against the resistance. Repeat on the other side.

Core (Obliques): Exercise: Seated Russian Twists

Description: Sit on the floor with knees bent and feet flat. Lean back slightly and twist your torso to one side, then the other. Hold a weight or keep hands together for increased resistance.

Hips (Hip Flexors): Exercise: Hip Flexor Stretch Description: Kneel on one knee with the other foot in front, producing a 90-degree angle. Shift your weight forward, feeling a stretch in the hip of the kneeling leg. Hold and exchange legs.

Balance and Stability (Entire Body): Exercise: Balancing on One Leg with Arm Raises

Description: Stand on one leg and elevate the other arm to shoulder height. Hold the position, then switch to the opposite leg and arm. This exercise increases overall balance and stability.

SETS AND REPS FOR EACH EXERCISE

Legs (Quadriceps, Hamstrings, Calves):

Exercise: Bodyweight Squats

Sets: 2-3 sets

Repetitions: 10-15 reps per set

Arms (Biceps, Triceps):

Exercise: Bicep Curls with Light Weights

Sets: 2 sets

Repetitions: 10-12 reps per set

Chest (Pectoral Muscles):

Exercise: Wall Push-Ups

Sets: 2-3 sets

Repetitions: 8-12 reps per set

Back (Latissimus Dorsi):

Exercise: Seated Rows with Resistance Band

Sets: 2 sets

Repetitions: 10-15 reps per set

Shoulders (Deltoids):

Exercise: Lateral Raises with Light Weights

Sets: 2 sets

Repetitions: 10-12 reps per set

Core (Abdominals, Lower Back):

Exercise: Seated Leg Lifts

Sets: 2-3 sets

Repetitions: 12-15 reps per set

Hips (Glutes):

Exercise: Glute Bridges
Sets: 2-3 sets
Repetitions: 10-12 reps per set
Balance (Legs, Core):

Exercise: One-Leg Stand
Sets: 2 sets
Repetitions: 20-30 seconds per leg
Legs (Quadriceps, Hamstrings, Calves):

Exercise: Standing Calf Raises
Sets: 2-3 sets
Repetitions: 12-15 reps per set
Arms (Forearms, Grip Strength):

Exercise: Forearm Squeezes with a Stress Ball
Sets: 2 sets
Repetitions: 15-20 reps per set
Chest (Pectoral Muscles):

Exercise: Chest Press with Resistance Band
Sets: 2 sets
Repetitions: 10-12 reps per set
Back (Rhomboids):

Exercise: Seated Band Pull-Apart
Sets: 2 sets

Repetitions: 12-15 reps per set
Shoulders (Rotator Cuff):

Exercise: Rotator Cuff External Rotation
Sets: 2 sets
Repetitions: 10-12 reps per set
Core (Obliques):

Exercise: Seated Russian Twists
Sets: 2-3 sets
Repetitions: 12-15 reps per set
Hips (Hip Flexors):

Exercise: Hip Flexor Stretch
Sets: 2 sets
Hold Time: 20-30 seconds per leg
Balance and Stability (Entire Body):

Exercise: Balancing on One Leg with Arm Raises
Sets: 2 sets
Repetitions: 10-12 reps per leg

Chapter 4

Enhancing Flexibility

IMPORTANCE OF FLEXIBILITY FOR SENIORS

In the tapestry of aging, the significance of flexibility for seniors unfurls as a fundamental cornerstone, not only confined to physical prowess but as an intricate weave of benefits that permeate the very fabric of a vibrant and meaningful life.

Preserving Unrestricted Mobility and Independence: Flexibility stands as the sentinel at the gates of mobility, preserving the ability to move with uncontrolled freedom and independence. For seniors, the power to smoothly reach, bend, and twist is not simply a physical attribute but a crucial key unlocking doors to prolonged self-sufficiency.

minimizing the Wear of Time on Joints: As joints weather the sands of time, flexibility exercises function as a gentle counterforce, staunchly lubricating the joints and minimizing the stiffness that can accompany the aging process. By embracing flexibility, elders engage in a proactive strategy to keeping a supple range of motion and avoiding discomfort.

Elevating Balance and Coordination to Zenith: A limber body is a balanced body. Flexibility assumes a crucial function in fortifying stability and coordination, so greatly minimizing the danger of falls. Seniors, by embracing activities that increase flexibility, build their base, allowing for confident movement and an elevated sense of stability.

Alleviating Discomfort and Championing Joint Health: Gentle stretches and flexibility exercises materialize as therapeutic cures, bringing respite from the inevitable aches and pains that may emerge with age. This is not only about physical comfort; it's a journey toward cultivating joint health, where flexibility becomes a soothing balm for the body.

Cultivating Mental Serenity Through Physical Harmony: The combination of body and mind in the pursuit of flexibility becomes an exquisite type of meditation. Accompanied by attentive breathing and intentional movements, flexibility exercises cultivate mental well-being, functioning as a salve to alleviate stress, anxiety, and cultivating a calm and concentrated state of mind.

Optimizing Circulation and Igniting Vitality: Like a soothing symphony orchestrating life's essence, flexibility exercises optimize blood circulation throughout the body. Improved blood flow means each cell receives its share of oxygen and nutrients, resulting in a heightened sensation of vitality that infuses seniors with fresh energy and a zest for life.

Fostering Social Bonds and Community Engagement: The pursuit of flexibility often evolves into social activity. Participating in group yoga courses or joining stretching sessions provides a conduit for social relationships. These shared experiences not only contribute to physical well-being but also generate channels for creating connections and a sense of community.

Embracing Aging with Positivity and Grace: Embracing flexibility exceeds a mere physical regimen; it is a declaration that aging is not a constraint but a constant evolution. Seniors who prioritize flexibility exercises typically find themselves adopting a positive view on aging. Each stretch becomes a conscious step toward a more fulfilling and active existence.

STRETCHING ROUTINES FOR IMPROVED FLEXIBILITY

In the search of greater flexibility for seniors, a careful and well-rounded stretching program becomes the compass directing the way. These carefully crafted stretches are designed to target major muscle groups, enhance joint mobility, and foster a profound sense of physical well-being. Remember to start cautiously, breathe slowly, and never force your body beyond its comfortable range.

Warm-Up: Gentle Joint Mobilization Neck Circles:

Slowly rotate your head in a circular manner, first clockwise, then counterclockwise.

Repeat 5 times in each direction.

Shoulder Rolls:

Lift your shoulders up towards your ears, then roll them back and down.

Repeat 10 times, then reverse the direction.

Wrist Circles:

Extend your arms in front and rotate your wrists in circular motions.

Repeat 8 times in each direction.

Ankle Alphabet:

Lift one foot and write the alphabet with your toes in the air.

Repeat with the other foot.

Lower Body Stretches:

Seated Forward Fold:

Sit with legs extended, reach toward your toes, maintaining your back straight.

Hold for 15-30 seconds.

Quad Stretch:

Stand or grab onto a chair for balance, bring one heel towards your buttocks.

Hold your ankle with your hand and gently press your hip forward.

Hold for 15-30 seconds on each leg.

Inner Thigh Stretch:

Sit with your back straight, soles of feet together, and slowly press your knees towards the floor.

Hold for 15-30 seconds.

Upper Body Stretches:

Triceps Stretch:

Raise one arm overhead, bend your elbow, and reach down your back.

Gently push on the bent elbow with your opposing hand.

Hold for 15-30 seconds on each arm.

Chest Opener:

Clasp your hands behind your back, straighten your arms, and elevate them slightly.

Open your chest and hold for 15-30 seconds.

Spine & Back Stretches:

Cat-Cow Stretch:

On hands and knees, arch your back upward (cat), then dip it down (cow).

Repeat for 1 minute.

Seated Spinal Twist:

Sit with legs outstretched, cross one leg over the other, and twist towards the bent knee.

Hold for 15-30 seconds on each side.

Flexibility and Balance Exercises:

Tree Pose:

Stand on one leg, place the sole of the other foot on the inner thigh or calf.

Hold for 30 seconds on each leg.

Heel-to-Toe Walk:

Walk in a straight line, placing the heel of one foot directly in front of the toes of the other.

Repeat for 10 steps.

Cool Down: Deep Breathing and Relaxation

Deep Belly Breathing:

Sit comfortable, inhale deeply through your nose, expanding your belly.

Exhale slowly through your mouth.

Repeat for 3-5 minutes.

Corpse Pose (Savasana):

Lie on your back, arms at your sides, palms facing up.

Close your eyes and focus on your breath, relaxing your entire body.

Hold for 5-10 minutes.

Lower Body Stretches: Hip Flexor Stretch:

Kneel on one knee, with the other foot in front, producing a 90-degree angle.

Gently push your hips forward, feeling the stretch at the front of your hip.

Hold for 15-30 seconds on each leg.

Calf Stretch:

Stand facing a wall, place your hands on the wall, and walk one foot back.

Keep the rear leg straight, heel on the ground, and softly lean forward.

Hold for 15-30 seconds on each leg.

Hamstring Stretch:

Sit with one leg outstretched and the sole of the other foot against the inner thigh.

Reach forward toward your toes, keeping your back straight.

Hold for 15-30 seconds on each leg.

Upper Body Stretches:

Neck Stretch:

Tilt your head to one side, moving your ear nearer your shoulder.

Hold for 15-30 seconds, then switch sides.

Upper Back Stretch:

Sit or stand with your feet shoulder-width apart, clasp your hands in front, and circle your back, extending forward.

Hold for 15-30 seconds.

Spine & Back Stretches:

Child's Pose:

Kneel on the floor, sit back on your heels, and reach your arms forward.

Hold for 30 seconds, feeling the stretch down your back.

Seated Forward Bend:

Sit with legs outstretched, hinge at your hips, and reach toward your toes.

Hold for 15-30 seconds, feeling the stretch in your lower back and hamstrings.

Flexibility and Balance Exercises:

Leg Swings:

Hold onto a firm surface, swing one leg forward and backward, then side to side.

Repeat for 10 swings on each leg.

Chair Leg Raises:

Sit in a firm chair, straighten one leg, hold for a few seconds, then drop it back down.

Repeat for 10 raises on each leg.

Cool Down: Deep Breathing and Relaxation

Seated Side Stretch:

Sit with knees crossed, extend one arm overhead, and slowly lean to the opposing side.

Hold for 15-30 seconds on each side.

Breathing Exercise with Arm Movement:

Inhale, raising your arms aloft, and exhale, lowering them back down.

Repeat for 3-5 minutes, synchronizing breath with movement.

CHAPTER 5

Holistic Workouts

Mind-Body Connection in Senior Fitness

In the area of senior fitness, the interwoven dance of the mind and body emerges as a meaningful path toward complete well-being. Beyond the realm of conventional physical exercise, this trip dives into the delicate tapestry of intentional motions, mindful workouts, and a heightened awareness of the symbiotic interaction between mental and physical aspects. In this inquiry, seniors embark on a transforming experience where the mind and body are not different entities but coalescent companions, co-creating a symphony of energy and wellness.

Embarking on Mindful Movement: Yoga and Tai Chi:

Mindful movement begins with practices like yoga and Tai Chi, which serve as conduits for the convergence of breath and motion. Seniors engaged in these disciplines find themselves fully present in each pose, cultivating mental clarity while gently nurturing physical strength and flexibility. The deliberate, intentional nature of these exercises builds a connection that extends beyond the physical sphere, diving into the realms of awareness and conscious embodiment.

Slow, Controlled activities: The technique of conscious movement extends to including intentional, slow-paced activities into the workout program. Whether it's regulated resistance exercise or focused stretches, seniors are taught to focus on the feelings within their bodies. This intentional technique produces a heightened awareness of muscle engagement, joint mobility, and the fluidity of movement. Through purposeful, controlled actions, seniors integrate their mental focus with the subtleties of physical motion.

Breath as the Bridge: Conscious Breathing Exercises:
At the center of the mind-body relationship resides the breath—a powerful bridge bridging the internal and outward realms. Conscious breathing exercises, such as diaphragmatic or rhythmic breathing, become fundamental components of senior fitness programs. These techniques synchronize the breath with movement, not only boosting oxygen flow but also developing a sense of calm and concentrated presence. The rhythmic ebb and flow of breath become a contemplative anchor, grounding seniors in the present moment.

Mindful Meditation: Mindful meditation, weaved smoothly into workout regimens, serves as a sanctuary for the mind. Whether in a seated position or during a quiet lying session, seniors are asked to devote their attention inward. This intentional concentration on breath and inner silence produces a serene state of mind, producing a mental space that compliments the physical rejuvenation attained via exercise.

Positive Visualization: Visualizing Success:

Harnessing the power of the mind, seniors are urged to engage in positive visualization as a vital part of their fitness path. Visualization techniques entail mentally rehearsing the completion of exercises or the achievement of specific fitness goals. This not only improves confidence but also generates a mental blueprint that the body can follow during physical activity, connecting the mind's vision with the body's capabilities.

Affirmations: Affirmations function as transforming mantras, altering the mental landscape of seniors engaged in fitness regimens. Positive affirmations, repeated consciously during exercise sessions, strengthen their skills and build a positive mindset. These affirmations become anchors, rooting seniors in a belief system that transcends physical constraints, inspiring them to reach new heights in their exercise efforts.

Sensory Engagement: Nature Walks and Outdoor Activities: Seniors are urged to activate their senses during outdoor activities, increasing the mind-body link. Whether it's a leisurely nature walk or gentle outdoor activities, the sights, sounds, and sensations of the environment heighten consciousness. The connection with nature becomes a sensory journey, immersing elders in the present moment and increasing the entire exercise experience.

Music Therapy: Incorporating music into training programs increases the sensory experience. Music has the unique capacity to elicit emotions and enrich the exercise process. Seniors find themselves moving in tune with the songs, producing a wonderful synthesis of physical and auditory stimulation. Music becomes a motivational force, boosting the mind-body connection and infusing the training program with joy and passion.

Mindful Hydration and Nutrition: Conscious Eating Practices:
Seniors are urged to approach meals with awareness, changing the act of eating into a sensory experience. By paying attention to the colors, textures, and flavors of food, they enrich the whole eating experience. This attentiveness not only improves healthy eating habits but also enhances the connection between sustenance and general well-being.

Hydration Rituals: Hydrating the body becomes a deliberate ritual rather than a routine activity. Seniors are urged to focus on the act of drinking water, savoring each sip, and noting the restoring effect it has on both body and mind. This intentional approach to hydration converts a basic physiological necessity into a conscious act of self-care.

Celebrating Progress: Gratitude Practice:
The practice of appreciation becomes a cornerstone of recognizing achievement in senior fitness. Seniors are encouraged to show thanks for the possibilities of their bodies. Recognizing and appreciating the power,

flexibility, and resilience displayed during each exercise session builds a good relationship with their physical self. Gratitude becomes a motivator for inspiration and a source of delight in the fitness path.

reflecting Journaling: Maintaining a fitness diary becomes a reflecting exercise, allowing seniors a space to capture their thoughts and experiences. Journaling provides an opportunity to connect with emotions, track progress, and celebrate achievements. As seniors put pen to paper, they build a narrative of their fitness journey

Integrating Yoga and Meditation

As individuals enter their elderly years, the emphasis on obtaining holistic well-being becomes increasingly significant. In this quest, the inclusion of both yoga and meditation takes on a key function as a catalyst for transformation. This strong combination provides seniors with a comprehensive approach to health, stretching beyond simply physical exercise to cover cerebral clarity, emotional equilibrium, and spiritual connection. In the orchestration of a holistic workout, the merger of yoga and meditation becomes an elegant composition, building a special and individualized trip that supports the well-being of the mind, body, and spirit.

The Foundations of Yoga for Seniors: Gentle Asanas and Movement:

Yoga, sometimes misconceived as a practice reserved for the young and flexible, is beautifully adapted to fulfill the demands of elders. Gentle asanas (poses) and attentive movements constitute the cornerstone of senior-friendly yoga. These postures prioritize accessibility, emphasizing comfort and alignment over intricacy. Seniors engage in movements that increase flexibility, balance, and joint health, producing a sense of refreshment in each pose.

Breath-Centered Practice: At the heart of yoga is the breath, and for seniors, cultivating a breath-centered practice is paramount. Pranayama, or breath control exercises, becomes a vital component. Techniques such as diaphragmatic breathing and alternate nostril breathing enhance respiratory function, induce relaxation, and serve as a bridge between the physical and mental components of well-being.

Adaptable Yoga Sequences for Seniors: Chair Yoga:
Recognizing that mobility could differ among seniors, chair yoga offers a sat option that doesn't compromise the benefits of traditional yoga. Seated postures, gentle stretches, and reduced motions accommodate varying fitness levels, making yoga inclusive for seniors with diverse abilities. Chair yoga provides an accessible channel for persons with restricted mobility or those who prefer a seated practice.

Standing postures with Support: For seniors desiring a standing practice, modified standing postures with the support of a chair or wall promote balance and stability. These postures are designed to build leg strength, enhance posture, and boost confidence in weight-bearing positions. The use of props, such as blocks or straps, enables a safe and supportive yoga practice.

The Mindful Journey of Meditation: Guided Meditation for

Relaxation:

Complementing the physicality of yoga, meditation becomes a gentle guide to inner calm. Guided meditation courses geared for elders focus on relaxation and stress reduction. Visualization techniques, soothing imagery, and mindfulness prompts create a serene setting, allowing seniors to unwind and center themselves despite the rush of life.

Mindfulness Meditation for Everyday Presence: Incorporating mindfulness meditation into the comprehensive workout program encourages seniors to embrace the skill of being present. Mindfulness practices entail devoting non-judgmental attention to the present moment. Seniors learn to examine ideas, sensations, and emotions without attachment, generating a sense of clarity, acceptance, and tranquility in their daily lives.

The Intersection of Yoga and Meditation: Mindful Movement in Yoga:

Yoga, when practiced thoughtfully, easily turns into a moving meditation. The rhythmic flow of asanas linked with focused breathwork generates a contemplative experience. Seniors find themselves fully absorbed in the present moment, establishing a mind-body connection that transcends the bounds of the yoga mat.

Savasana (Corpse Pose) and Meditation Integration: Every yoga practice closes with Savasana, a pose of rest and integration. This transition serves as a gateway to meditation. Guided relaxation and breath awareness during Savasana gently transfer elders into a contemplative state. The seamless transition from the energetic practice of yoga to the calm of meditation reflects the holistic nature of the combined approach.

Holistic Benefits for Seniors: Physical Well-Being:

The physical benefits of mixing yoga and meditation are abundant for seniors. Increased flexibility, increased balance, enhanced joint mobility, and better posture contribute to overall physical well-being. Yoga's gentle nature corresponds with the principles of aging gracefully, boosting strength and energy without unnecessary strain.

Cognitive and Emotional Health: The harmony of yoga and meditation extends beyond the physical, embracing cognitive and emotional worlds. Mindful movement and meditation techniques have been connected to cognitive function improvement, memory enhancement, and stress reduction. Seniors enjoy a mental clarity that transcends the mat, positively benefiting daily life.

Social Connection and Community: Group yoga and meditation sessions develop a sense of community and social connection among elders. Shared experiences, supportive environments, and the camaraderie created in these sessions add to a comprehensive feeling of well-being. The community aspect boosts the total impact of the holistic workout, creating an inclusive space for elders to thrive.

Empowering Seniors on Their Holistic Journey: Tailored Instruction and Modifications:

Recognizing the individuality of each senior's body and abilities, tailored teaching and changes are important. Instructors experienced in teaching elders through yoga and meditation modify practices to individual needs. This tailored approach guarantees that each senior obtains the entire spectrum of advantages while respecting their physical limits.

Encouraging Consistency and Regular Practice: Consistency is crucial to receiving the full effects of a holistic workout. Encouraging elders to include yoga and meditation into their routine promotes a sense of commitment to their well-being. Whether done everyday or a few times a week, a consistent habit boosts the cumulative effects, encouraging prolonged physical, mental, and emotional wellness.

CHAPTER 6:

Staying Motivated

Overcoming Challenges

Seniors facing many challenges as they lose weight and gain flexibility must be motivated and resilient. Maintaining a fun and lasting workout regimen requires acknowledging and resolving these issues. This comprehensive book will cover frequent issues elders experience and offer practical solutions to overcome them and succeed in exercise.

Understanding Senior Fitness: Living in the golden years involves considerable changes in priorities, skills, and perspectives. These adjustments can help and hinder seniors' weight loss and flexibility fitness journeys. Representing this demographic's different experiences and tailoring fitness strategies to individual needs is crucial.

1. Accepting Physical Limits:

Challenge:

Arthritis and diminished mobility can make certain workouts difficult and frustrating for seniors.

Our strategy is to tailor our approach to each individual's needs and talents. Low-impact sports such as swimming or walking are soft on joints, leading to weight loss without putting unnecessary stress on the body. Additionally, chair yoga can deliver the benefits of traditional yoga in a seated position, making it accessible to those with mobility limitations.

2. Dealing with Fluctuating Energy Levels:

Challenge:

Energy levels among seniors can fluctuate, reducing their motivation for regular activity. Finding the drive to engage in a workout can be tough, particularly during periods of low energy.

Strategy: Understanding the patterns of energy swings is key. Planning workouts during times of the day when energy levels are naturally higher can make a major difference. Breaking down workouts into shorter, more manageable sessions throughout the day encourages seniors to keep active without feeling overwhelmed. Additionally, including things they enjoy can enhance motivation, turning exercise into a source of rejuvenation rather than tiredness.

3. Finding Variety in Workouts:

Challenge: Monotonous habits can lead to boredom, lowering

motivation over time.

Strategy: Injecting variation into the training program is vital for keeping things fresh and engaging. This can include alternating between different sorts of activities such as aerobic workouts, weight training, and flexibility exercises. Exploring new activities or attending group classes offers an aspect of socialization and enjoyment, making the overall experience more gratifying.

4. Setting Realistic and Attainable Goals:

Challenge: Setting overly ambitious goals that are tough to fulfill might lead to dissatisfaction and a sense of failure.

Strategy: Establishing realistic and progressive goals is crucial. Celebrate minor victories along the road, whether it's completing a specified amount of steps, developing flexibility, or regularly following to a training plan for a specific length. This strategy not only promotes confidence but also gives a path for continual growth.

5. Maintaining Consistency: struggle: Consistency is commonly recognized as a struggle, especially when facing disruptions such as travel or unanticipated health issues.

Strategy: Developing a flexible routine that can adjust to varied circumstances is key. Incorporating exercises that may be done at home or while traveling ensures that fitness remains a continuous component of the senior's lifestyle. Consistency is not about perfection but about making consistent, lasting efforts towards the overarching fitness goals.

6. Overcoming Psychological Barriers: Challenge: Psychological

barriers, like self-doubt and fear of damage, can inhibit progress.

Strategy: Cultivating a positive mindset is vital for overcoming psychological limitations. Focus on the benefits of exercise, both physical and mental. Engage in activities that improve mental well-being, such as meditation or mindfulness techniques. Seeking support from friends, family, or a fitness group can bring encouragement and a sense of togetherness.

7. Making Fitness a Social Activity: Challenge: Isolation can contribute to lost motivation and a lack of accountability.

Strategy: Turning fitness into a social pursuit addresses the difficulty of isolation. Exercising with friends, joining group classes, or participating in community events gives a social element to the fitness routine. Shared experiences and the encouragement of peers form a supportive network that promotes motivation and enjoyment.

8. Seeking Professional Guidance: Challenge: Navigating the fitness road alone can be intimidating, especially when considering specific health concerns.

Strategy: Seeking professional help from healthcare specialists or trained fitness coaches is crucial. These professionals can provide individualized guidance, taking into consideration particular health issues and limits. A personalized approach ensures that workouts are safe, effective, and connected with the senior's overall well-being.

9. Incorporating Enjoyable things: Challenge: Forcing oneself to engage in things that are not enjoyable might lead to boredom and a lack of motivation.

Strategy: Selecting tasks that bring joy and fulfillment is vital for maintaining long-term motivation. Whether it's dancing, gardening, or participating in recreational sports, finding delight in the workout contributes to maintained engagement. The goal is to make fitness an enjoyable and gratifying experience.

10. Tracking Progress: Challenge: A lack of apparent progress may demotivate elders, forcing them to question the efficacy of their efforts.

Strategy: Keeping a fitness notebook is a powerful tool for tracking improvement. Documenting achievements, improvements, and even problems offers a visual record of the positive impact of constant work. Reflecting on these entries reinforces the sense that every step, no matter how tiny, adds to total advancement.

CELEBRATING MILESTONES

As we grow older, going on a fitness journey tailored to weight loss, strength growth, and greater flexibility marks a praiseworthy quest necessary for enhancing well-being in our later years. Within this transformative endeavor aimed at improving physical health and quality of life, the simple yet profound act of celebrating milestones along the way becomes a pivotal cornerstone, essential for sustaining motivation, cultivating positivity, and fully recognizing the substantial strides made on the winding path to a healthier, more active, and more resilient lifestyle.

The path begins with the formulation of individualized, attainable goals that coincide with our own fitness aspirations and present capabilities. Setting customized objectives geared to our specific needs and current fitness level allows us to design a course that is both suitably challenging and realistically feasible. These goals serve as a roadmap, providing direction and helping break down a massive endeavor into digestible steps.

As we strive towards these goals, accepting and finding joy in little, incremental wins and victories generates an encouraging attitude of constant growth. Each modest win, whether it be walking for five minutes longer than the day before or lifting slightly larger weights than last week, acts as a small building block, contributing to our overall sense of good progress and personal accomplishment. Recognizing these little yet meaningful achievements provides regular bursts of encouragement that propel us ahead.

Likewise, appreciating concrete advances in our physical health and talents earned through exercise immediately reinforces the significant impact regular fitness can have on our bodies at any age. These achievements are a monument to the extraordinary durability and adaptability of the human body, illustrating the transforming benefits constant effort and dedication can have on our strength, endurance, mobility, balance, cardiovascular health, and general physical well-being. They are reminders that growth is certainly attainable through commitment.

Just as essential as physical feats are the modest behavioral adjustments that often follow a new fitness plan. Milestones in this realm include accomplishing regular workout schedules, increasing workout duration, keeping discipline on rest days, improving diet, increasing water intake, and more. These modifications stress our ability to establish and stick to sustainable, healthy habits at every stage of life, laying the foundation for long-term well-being.

On a broader level, the practice of celebrating little successes supports the growth of a happy outlook. It emphasizes the notion that each and every step forward in our fitness path, no matter how tiny it may seem, constitutes a big triumph deserving of credit and celebration. This mentality in turn bolsters our feeling of self-confidence and resilience, arming us with a "can-do" attitude to persist in the face of hardship.

On a practical level, employing tools like milestone calendars, charts, or journals to document and physically reflect our progress provides as a continuing source of inspirational motivation. Having a concrete record of accomplishments and being able to literally see marks of development across weeks and months is an illuminating reminder of how far we've gone. These diaries become living testimony of our journey's evolution.

Additionally, sharing milestones and joys with friends, family, or a wider fitness group adds a social component that may greatly improve the experience. Positive appreciation and encouragement from loved ones helps foster a sense of community celebration and accountability. It magnifies the value of achievements by allowing others to join in the joy and meaning of our journey.

Likewise, building a personal reward system related to attaining milestones can further stimulate our efforts by providing an element of excitement and positive reinforcement. Having modest pleasures to look forward to, like a soothing massage, great dinner out, purchase of something special, or any other pleasurable activity, offers us something to aim towards. The sense of anticipation fundamental to working towards a reward contributes to the overall happiness and satisfaction of our fitness journey.

Carving out time for regular reflection also allows us to fully grasp the substantial yet complex growth of our fitness attitude and habits over weeks, months, and years. Taking stock of how far we've gone since initially lacing up those sneakers months or years ago develops sincere thankfulness for the progress gained thus far and drives ongoing dedication. Reflection provides perspective on all the struggles we've conquered and growth we've attained.

Once a milestone is accomplished, the quick formulation of new, incremental goals serves to maintain ongoing forward momentum and prevent complacency. Setting fresh fitness aims and challenges means our journey always feels dynamic, exciting, and full of potential rather than growing stale. There are always fresh frontiers to work for.

For lasting well-being, the ultimate milestone is effortlessly integrating regular exercise and deliberate healthy choices into the fabric of daily life rather than perceiving them as a separate task or short-term remedy. We want better fitness to become an intrinsic pillar of our identity and values moving forward. Celebrating milestones is most meaningful when they encourage this complete lifestyle adjustment.

Customizing exactly how we commemorate milestone achievements to match with personal preferences can considerably improve the importance of each win. We can celebrate through social gatherings, serious musings, personal words of congratulations, sharing images of progress online, enjoyment of a great meal, booking a needed massage, or any number of activities meaningful to us. The options are infinite.

Likewise, consistency itself deserves attention as a major achievement. Diligently sticking to a training regimen week after week indicates significant attention to our long-term well-being. After all, it is the modest choices made day in and day out that pave the way to substantial transformation. Recognizing the great worth of patient, continuous effort fosters motivation.

In addition to concrete indicators like weight lost or inches gone, noting and commemorating non-scale accomplishments is vital too. Improved energy levels, attitude, self-confidence, sleep quality, mental clarity, and lessened aches and pains are all tremendously crucial achievements worth celebrating. These speak to better inner wellness and quality of life.

Finally, deliberately establishing a strong support system among family, friends, or a wider community that wants to actively engage in celebrating your achievements along the way generates a priceless social ecology of encouragement. Their engagement enhances motivation and joy threefold. Knowing others are rooting for our success and identify with the significance of each victory makes the journey much more joyful and sustainable. We all need cheerleaders.

The path to greater fitness and wellbeing in our later years is surely a twisting road fraught with hurdles. However, by developing a patient, compassionate mindset focused on celebrating minor "wins" along the road, we may turn exercise from scary duty to joyous experience. With the appropriate mindset focused on progress over perfection, each milestone achievement, no matter how tiny it may appear, puts us one step closer to becoming our healthiest, most active selves. The key is recognizing and delighting in each minor accomplishment. In aggregate, they offer a rewarding road to greater well-being.

Chapter 7

Safety Considerations

Tips for Exercising Safely as a Senior

As we grow older, maintaining an active lifestyle becomes increasingly crucial for preserving our health, independence, and general wellness. Regular physical activity offers a plethora of benefits for seniors, including increasing cardiovascular health, maintaining bone density, reducing joint stiffness, preventing muscle loss, elevating mood, and reducing the risk of chronic illnesses including heart disease, diabetes, and osteoporosis. However, while exercise is incredibly helpful, safety should be the foremost consideration for older folks when embarking on any fitness plan. Caution and diligent care must be used to prevent preventable injuries. This thorough guide provides critical recommendations for exercising properly as a senior, ensuring you get the plentiful pleasures of physical activity while limiting unnecessary danger.

Before diving into specifics, it is vital to fully appreciate the varied value of fitness in our latter years. Strength training, cardiovascular exercise, flexibility training and balancing exercises all play key roles in maintaining muscle mass, bone density, joint mobility, response time, coordination, and total functional independence. Physically, being active keeps our cardiovascular system, lungs, and circulatory system healthy while preventing the muscle loss and stiffness that commonly accompanies aging. Just as significant, exercise helps prevent cognitive decline and emotional disorders including anxiety, despair and mood swings. Both the physical and mental health benefits significantly promote continuing healthiness and a great quality of life throughout our elderly years. Given these wide-ranging benefits, exercising frequently should be a lifelong priority. However, preserving safety should be the number one issue while creating your training regimen.

The following guidelines provide helpful advise on exercising properly as you age:

Before beginning any new workout program, even if you have exercised before, it is wise to consult your physician or healthcare professional. Outline your fitness goals and discuss your present state of health. A full medical assessment can reveal any pre-existing conditions or limits that may necessitate adaptations to your fitness regimen or special precautions to take. This is a very crucial first step for managing chronic conditions.

When creating your routine, emphasize low-impact workouts that reduce excessive strain on the joints. Activities like walking, swimming, cycling, and rowing machines provide excellent cardiovascular benefits while being mild on joints. Conversely, high-impact workouts like sprinting and jumping can worsen joint pain and are best avoided.

Allot time before your primary workout to warm-up appropriately. Warm-up exercises like light cardio, dynamic stretches, and joint rotations stimulate blood flow to the muscles, improve range of motion, increase core body temperature and prepare the body for more intensive exertion. A cautious warm-up prevents injury.

Incorporate strength training into your schedule two to three times each week. Light weight training preserves and grows muscle mass while supporting joint, bone and ligament health. Using free weights, resistance bands, or weight machines, focus on major muscle groups. Build up steadily over time.

Include balance exercises like heel-to-toe walking, standing on one foot, and tai chi to refine stability and minimize falls, which grow increasingly common as we age. These exercises strengthen the muscles supporting joints, increase core strength, and enhance general coordination. Regular practice is crucial.

Stay well hydrated before, during and after exercise. Drink plenty of water, even if not feeling thirsty. Dehydration exacerbates muscle cramps, disorientation, and heat-related diseases. Hydration is crucial during physical exertion.

Listen attention to your body throughout each workout. Immediately halt any exercise generating sudden joint swelling, soreness or discomfort surpassing usual exertion. Seek medical advice when needed. Differentiating normal discomfort from potential harm is crucial.

Use suitable, well-fitted footwear and equipment for your chosen activity to support joints and muscles while minimizing errors. Proper running or walking shoes are a smart investment for basic activity. Yoga mats provide traction and stability during floor workouts.

For seniors who are new to exercising or resuming after an extended layoff, progress gradually to enable your body time to adjust to greater demands. Avoid the tendency to push too hard too soon, which often leads to sprains, strains and exhaustion. Build up duration and intensity slowly.

Incorporate flexibility training like yoga, static stretching, and range of motion exercises to preserve joint health and mobility. Dynamic stretches before cardiac activities warm up muscles, while holding static stretches after workouts promotes total flexibility.

Maintain good posture and technique throughout exercise to avoid pressure on the spine and joints. Engage core muscles to support the back. Stand tall. Whether performing squats, crunches, or bicep curls, regulated technique reduces damage.

Consider joining senior-tailored fitness courses which give adequately paced, low-impact activities under an instructor's instruction. Group lessons also give incentive and fellowship. Explore offerings at local community centers.

Get your heart pounding several times a week through cardiac exercise. Brisk walking, swimming, cycling, or low-impact aerobics sessions boost heart rate for extended periods, supporting cardiovascular health. Aim for at least 150 minutes of moderate-intensity cardio each week with rest days.

When exercising outdoors, carefully consider environmental variables including heat, humidity, wind chill and sun exposure which might effect older adults more dramatically. Exercise in the chill of morning or evening. In winter, dress warmly and careful of slick surfaces.

Allow adequate time between sessions for full muscle recovery. Scheduling frequent rest days minimizes overtraining which can lead to injury and exhaustion. Recovery permits muscles to heal and strengthen.

The path to safe, successful and pleasurable exercise as a senior is available to those prepared to take the appropriate safeguards. Consult your doctor, progress cautiously, listen to your body attentively, use adequate gear, and vary your routine to include aerobic, strength training, flexibility and balancing elements. With sufficient care, exercise can substantially strengthen bodily and mental health while accommodating illnesses such as arthritis, osteoporosis and joint pain. A tailored fitness plan promotes vitality, energy and engagement with life. Staying active adds immensely to good aging.

Common Mistakes to Avoid

Embarking on a fitness adventure in our later years can seem scary, but with correct care, it can also be tremendously rewarding. Avoiding frequent mistakes is key to having a safe, effective, and pleasurable fitness regimen. Being aware of these potential problems allows us to consciously create activities that enhance health and limit harm risks. With attentive planning, elders can construct uplifting workout regimes that boost quality of life. Here are some significant mistakes to be cautious of when exercising beyond 50:

One of the most typical blunders is omitting to adequately warm-up before jumping into rigorous activity or cool down afterwards. Jumping immediately into high-intensity training can strain muscles and tendons, boosting the possibility of pulls, tears and sprains. Cooling down with gentle aerobics and full-body stretches post-workout minimizes muscular stiffness and pain by bringing nutrient-rich blood back into tissues. Gradually easing in and out of workout sessions promotes performance and improves recovery.

Likewise, focusing primarily on cardiovascular exercises while ignoring strength training is an overlook. Maintaining and developing muscle mass becomes increasingly critical as we age to support joint health, improve balance, preserve bone density, and sustain general mobility and functional independence. Using resistance bands, free weights, or weight machines 2-3 times a week reduces the muscle loss associated with aging. Aim for routines targeting all main muscle groups.

When strength training, adopting poor form is another typical problem. Lifting too rapidly or pushing through discomfort often leads to injury and poor training efficacy. Mastering regulated, precise motions by aligning joints and engaging core muscles should take priority over intensity. If uncertain about form, try working with a personal trainer when initially getting started. Proper technique prevents stresses.

Staying well hydrated during and after sweating is also vital. Forgetting to drink sufficient water while an exercise can result in dehydration, particularly on hot days. Dehydration causes muscle cramps, spasms, lightheadedness and exacerbates weariness. Drink water before, during and post-workout to restore fluids lost during activity. Additionally, listen attentively for indications from your body warning overexertion, such heavy breathing and strong thirst.

Pushing through intense pains or discomfort is an extra red indicator. While some muscular soreness is normal, intense discomfort suggests probable injury. Exercising through pain often worsens damage to joints or muscles. Instead, stop activities immediately and consult a physician if pain persists. Distinguishing normal muscle tiredness from signals of damage is crucial. The cliché "no pain, no gain" should not apply.

Setting unrealistic fitness ambitions might sometimes be damaging. Establishing overambitious goals sometimes leads to dissatisfaction and a sense of failure if not accomplished fast. This inhibits continued engagement. Set incremental, clear milestones appropriate with your present abilities and time commitments. Achievable milestones, like walking 10 minutes without tiredness or lifting 5-pound weights, provide mile markers of achievement.

Tailoring training intensity and duration to personal fitness levels is also crucial. Maintaining persistently high exertion as a novice increases injury risk and exhaustion. Honor your body's demands by altering exertion based on energy levels. Completing a lesser workout is preferable than leaving one from exhaustion. Build increasing intensity incrementally. Patience prevents harm.

Relying primarily on cardiovascular machines like ellipticals neglects the benefits of cross-training. Well-rounded fitness routines include strength training, flexibility exercises and balance work. While cardio strengthens the heart, merely utilizing these equipment long-term might imbalance overall fitness. Variety ensures all-encompassing health. Explore options like yoga, Pilates or swimming.

Relatedly, omitting to integrate balance and flexibility exercise is hazardous. Balance exercises like tandem stance and tai chi hone stability, reducing falls. Flexibility training such as yoga and stretching maintains range of motion and joint health. These become increasingly crucial for mobility as we age yet are often disregarded. Schedule time for both.

Just as vital is scheduling regular recovery days between

strengthening exercises. While consistency is vital, muscles require 48 hours minimum to heal and rebuild effectively. Overtraining through skipped rest days stresses muscles, often causing injury. Dedicate 1-2 rest days every week for optimal performance and improvement.

Seeking help from physical therapists, personal trainers or your physician when first getting started is also suggested. These professionals customize regimens specific to individual health problems and demands, lowering risk of consequences. Allowing ego to avoid professional consultation might be detrimental long-term. Be your own health champion.

Being conscious of indications from your body like pain, unexpected weariness and disorientation is crucial. Ignoring these warning signs and pushing through might change safe pain into harm. Always listen to your body first. Keeping a fitness journal helps uncover concerning habits.

Likewise, poor footwear raises injury risk. Supportive, well-fitted athletic shoes with enough traction assist prevent slips and falls when exercising. Replace sneakers after 300-500 miles. Proper footwear reduces pressure off joints. Don't ignore this vital gear.

Getting annual check-ups ensures your doctor assesses exercise safety given developing health considerations. Conditions like hypertension or osteoporosis may demand activity changes over time. Routine wellness checkups encourage healthy lifetime fitness engagement. Make these a priority.

For motivation, avoid continuously comparing your fitness progress to others. Getting discouraged by someone else's regimen reduces own accomplishments. Fitness is an individual journey. Comparing milestones with peers distracts from your inner wellness. Celebrate your own tiny gains.

Later-life exercise when undertaken wisely and listen to one's body increases health, independence and resilience. Sidestepping typical blunders minimizes risks of problems, enhancing safe participation. With excellent supervision and acceptable goals, elders can thrive via fitness. Mobility and vigor await individuals ready to learn basic safeguards and embrace their strongest selves.

Chapter 8

Real-Life Success Stories

Here are some inspirational stories of seniors reaching amazing heights through exercise and perseverance:

At age 56, Ernestine Shepherd went on a path to get healthy that converted her into a record-holding competitive female bodybuilder. After losing a bet to her sister, Ernestine began a weight training routine that astonishingly shaped her figure. Defying all odds, she joined and won bodybuilding competitions in her 70s and 80s, earning the Guinness World Record holder as the world's oldest competitive female bodybuilder. Ernestine illustrates that age is no barrier to accomplishing your objectives. Her unwavering desire pushes people to take charge of their health.

Charles Eugster similarly illustrates the great potential for physical fitness beyond our youth. After retiring at 65, Charles was disillusioned and lacked energy. So at age 87, he joined a local gym and began high-intensity strength and aerobic training. Over the next two decades, Charles molded an ideal body and went on to achieve many sprinting world records past age 95, including the 200-meter and 400-meter sprints. His credo that "age is just a number" pushes people to never stop achieving ambitious objectives.

At age 67, Ida Keeling discovered running as a means to deal with losing her two sons to drug-related violence just years apart. The catastrophic losses left her sad, however running offered serenity, regeneration and a new sense of purpose. She began exercising regularly and soon excelled in races. In her 100s, Ida established many sprint records, becoming the fastest woman in her age class. Despite terrible loss, Ida found consolation and courage through exercise, exemplifying the healing power of movement.

In her mid-30s, Yvonne Dowlen serendipitously found figure skating and instantly became fascinated. Though starting far later than most competitors, Yvonne improved to high-level talents via relentless work. She went on to captivate audiences with her beautiful acts for almost five decades. At age 80, she was still competing and performing around Europe. Yvonne symbolizes perseverance, demonstrating it's truly never too late to flourish at a new love.

Nicknamed the "Iron Nun," Sister Madonna Buder finished her first Ironman triathlon at age 52. Inspired by her pupils' triathlon training,

Sister Madonna found her own ability for rigorous endurance feats. She went on to finish almost 40 Ironman events between years 55 and 82, earning her the suitable title. A skilled swimmer, biker and runner, Sister Madonna illustrates the power of perseverance and drive to surpass limits.

At age 9, Johanna Quaas joined a local gymnastics club, setting the groundwork for a lifetime passion of the sport. Decades later, in her late 50s, Johanna returned to gymnastics and competitive competitions after raising her children. By her late 80s, she was still competing and executing gymnastic feats like handstands. Johanna, hailed as the World's Oldest Gymnast, highlighted the remarkable lifespan a good body and soul can bring. Her desire shines clearly.

Lew Hollander realized his ability for surviving physical obstacles after retirement. At age 82, Lew prepared relentlessly to realize his ambition of completing an Ironman Triathlon. Defying even his own expectations, Lew finished the tough 140-mile route in 16.5 hours, becoming the world's oldest Ironman at age 82. His tale emphasizes that we should never stop chasing our highest aspirations regardless of age. Anything is conceivable.

Jack LaLanne, renowned as the Godfather of Fitness, maintained an amazing fitness program until death at age 96. A pioneer in fitness and nutrition, Jack pushed strength training and good eating decades before its general appeal. His remarkable accomplishments like underwater jumping jacks and towing over 70 boats while chained and shackled displayed tremendous athleticism. Jack's lifelong passion and activism pushed millions to embrace fitness.

Despite life's obstacles and the passing decades, these folks illustrate the remarkable potential for our bodies and souls via exercise. Their determination, endurance and work ethic in chasing new tasks even into their senior years provide as strong encouragement. Age does not define restrictions. With enthusiasm and determination, tremendous achievements await. Their tales motivate and encourage us all.

CONCLUSION

Embarking on a fitness adventure in our later years offers huge promise to boost our health, energy, and quality of life as we age. However, in order to gain the varied advantages of exercise, it is vital that elders take certain precautions and follow expert counsel. A deliberate, holistic approach includes the physical, mental, emotional and social elements of wellness. Realistic goal-setting, sufficient nutrition, adequate rest, and injury avoidance should be stressed. Paying attentive attention to our body's cues is vital. While physical fitness is crucial, a positive mentality focused on progress over perfection is as key to keeping motivated. Patience, adaptation and recognizing minor successes pave the route to success. No matter our starting place, with proper care and commitment, we can all experience happy, vibrant and meaningful aging via exercise. The trip brings forth our strongest selves. If we take it one step at a time, improved health and wellbeing await.

Encouragement for Continued Fitness Journey

Here is some encouragement for continuing your fitness journey based on the important elements from the content:

The route to vitality and wellness via fitness in our older years might have its hurdles, but the rewards make it all worthwhile. Take satisfaction in how far you've gone already. Every step forward, no matter how tiny, symbolizes true progress. Don't become disheartened by setbacks. They are natural on any travel. Just continue your regimen as soon as you can. Your body will reward you for it.

Remember that this is your own route. Go at your own speed, listen to your body, and celebrate your personal successes. Comparing yourself to others serves no one. You have so much inner power, endurance and insight to tap into. Remind yourself daily why you started this path, and all the ways exercise brightens you up, inside and out.

Keep focused on feeling good in the current moment during each workout. The physical and mental clarity from regular action will continue accumulating in profoundly favorable ways. And you could just amaze yourself with what you can do. But even on challenging days, just showing up and doing what you can helps establish lifelong exercise habits.

Take joy in nourishing your health and wellbeing each day. You are giving your mind, body and spirit an essential service. Take time to absorb the fresh energy you feel. This is about so much more than physical looks. You are making an investment in your quality of life now and for many years to come. Be your own cheerleader, and believe that you have all you need inside you to attain your fitness objectives. Keep up the amazing job!

About the Author

Bailey Blake is a passionate advocate for healthy and active aging. As a fitness trainer and wellness coach specializing in senior fitness, Bailey has over 15 years of experience assisting older individuals uncover the joy and vibrancy that remaining active can bring to their lives.

Bailey's interest in geriatric fitness began early on while assisting at a retirement community gym during high school. Seeing firsthand the dramatic impact regular exercise had on residents' health and outlook inspired Bailey to learn everything possible about senior fitness. This motivation led Bailey to become a certified personal trainer and pursue ongoing education in areas like injury prevention, nutrition, and mindfulness for seniors.

Over the years, Bailey has worked with hundreds of seniors, listening to their needs and assisting tailor fitness regimens to match their lifestyles and capabilities. Bailey found great fulfillment in motivating older adults to realize they can accomplish remarkable fitness exploits through consistency and belief in themselves.

When not working one-on-one with clients, Bailey teaches specialized senior fitness classes and gives seminars on topics like holistic wellness, motivation, and overcoming setbacks on the fitness journey. Bailey also volunteers at a local senior center conducting chair yoga and calisthenics.

Through this book, Bailey wishes to empower as many seniors as possible to take control of their wellbeing. Bailey firmly believes vibrant aging is available to all willing to embrace exercise and healthy living on their own terms. Helping seniors live life to the utmost is Bailey's pleasure

Acknowledgments

I would like to express my sincerest appreciation to all those who helped make this book possible and contributed their insights and expertise.

Thank you to the inspiring seniors who shared their experiences, struggle,s and wisdom on the fitness journey. Your perseverance and passion for augmenting quality of life through activity even in your later years serves as a potent motivator.

I extend my gratitude to the physicians, trainers, physical therapists, and wellness professionals who offered invaluable guidance on safe exercise, injury prevention, goal-setting, and holistic health. Your specialized knowledge helps ensure seniors can undertake fitness regimens in ways that empower rather than overwhelm.

Thanks to the researchers and scientists whose work on exercise, aging, and geriatric wellness provided a foundation of evidence-based information. Your work illuminates the multifaceted advantages of remaining active and engaged.

I am grateful to the staff at senior centers and retirement communities who gave insights into establishing inclusive programs tailored to older adults' diverse needs and capabilities. You are assisting elder generations embrace the vibrancy of their years.

Finally, I sincerely salute my editors and colleagues whose feedback and collaboration helped refine and focus my vision. It is not always an easy road, but you gave me the courage to see it through.

This book was a collaborative endeavor to share essential, practical ways seniors can enrich their lives through holistic fitness. I hope it motivates and empowers elder individuals to pursue activity that fulfills both body and spirit. Here's to aging vibrantly on our own unique terms.